Homemade Herbal Hair Oil Infusions

Homemade Herbal Hair Oil Infusions

Easy Guide to Herbal Hair Oil Infusions Recipes for Hair Growth, Dry/Damaged Hair, Dandruff and Healthy Scalp

Tiffany Nicholas

Copyright

Disclaimer & Statement of Rights

Dedication

This guide is dedicated to those who have been looking for natural ways to take care of their hair and scalp.

TABLE OF CONTENTS

INTRODUCTION

Hair care products are moving from chemical-based ingredients towards all-natural boasting of herbal ingredients and essential oils. Herbal conditioners and shampoos promise to make hair shiny and healthy. No wonder the use of organic ingredients is the leading task in research and development of hair care products lately.

Sadly, natural-based hair care products are expensive. This is the main reason why we have to create herbal hair care product recipes that are affordable that can be done at home.

Although some people will swear that commercial hair products are more effective than the herbal, but they don't consider the disadvantages of commercial brands. Apart from the harsh chemicals used in making these commercial products, they produce more foam, leading to most of the problems associated with hair and scalp. However, herbal hair care recipes are made with herbs, essential oils, and water that will not make it foam as much as the commercial products.

Natural ingredients are much gentler on the hair and scalp. They will cleanse, shine, and make hair and scalp healthy. One of the options of natural hair care treatments is herbal hair infusion. This treatment will offer the benefits of organic herbs and natural oils to the hair and scalp.

Applying these oils into the hair will enhance the strands' strength and aids the improvement of the hair. The moment the oil is infused with herbs, there are added benefits that followed

each property of the herb that will help in the control of dandruff, management of early gray hair, treatment of scalp, nourishment of dry hair, and other hair and scalp problems.

This book is about all the following:

The advantages of organic-based products over chemical-based products.

How to create hair care treatment recipes using organic ingredients.

How to make your herbal hair care recipes that are affordable.

How to have healthy, shiny, long hair.

How to have a healthy scalp.

This book is your resource guide on how to DIY herbal hair infusion oil.

Chapter 1

HAIR CARE

Hair to us as human beings is a fundamental expression of the way we were created. No wonder when the hair is looking at its best, we always feel good and looking radiant. No matter how simple it is taking care of hair, we don't want to do it wrongly. Most times, it is not about how the products are being used, but the types of hair care products been used.

Recent surveys suggested that over 90% of women are not okay with the way their hair and are ready to trade it with sister, colleague, or friend. Some experts even suggested that apart from their eyes and smile, hair is another reason why most women get a good number of compliments.

Recent statistics show that the global haircare market in 2017 is around 85.5 billion US dollars, and the estimated future spending will be approximately 100 billion US dollars in 2023. Consumers are now looking for products that will take care of their hair with fewer chemicals on their hair. This change in orientation led to the popularity of herbal care treatments and products.

IMPORTANCE OF HAIR CARE

You don't have to be told how important to take good care of hair. It is your hair that makes you attractive or unattractive as the case may be. After smiles, flawless skin, and eyes, your hair plays a vital role in physical appearance.

The way you style your hair will portray so many things about you. If you are the type that always styles her hair regularly, your hair could be brittle and split.

Experience has shown that some hair care products can cause dryness and scalp itchiness because of the harsh chemical ingredients.

With some simple steps, you can reduce damages that these popular products may want to do on your hair:

Wash your hair regularly: Whenever you wash your hair, you must massage the scalp to keep it clean and healthy. Know that a clean scalp will make the hair healthy.

Choose the appropriate hair care: Most of the hair care products out there contain harsh chemicals that will damage hair. So the best advice is to use hair care products that contain natural-based ingredients.

Use of blow-dryer: If there is a need for you to use a blow-dryer, set it on low heat to reduce any damages, it may cause your hair.

Give hair a break: It is essential to give your hair a break at times. Don't use any hair care product on it for some time. Allow it to be natural.

Trim your hair: If you want your hair to look good and healthy, makes it a habit to trim it. Hair is just like a grass growing.

Feed your Hair: Your hair needs substances like vitamins, protein, and mineral-rich foods to thrive. These substances will help the hair to grow and develop.

Give hair hot oil treatment: If you want your hair to shine and be less prone to damage, give it hot oil treatments.

MOST COMMON HAIR ISSUES

Every woman would want their hair to be shiny, voluminous, and luscious, and achieving this feat can be a challenge. Having this kind of hair requires time, money, and appropriate maintenance. The typical hair problems can be a product of different types of factors that include environmental, genetic, chemical, and mechanical. Hair is exposed to several stresses throughout the day, and it can be challenging to bring them back to health and balance. The factors below are some of the most common hair issues:

Weak, Fine, and Lifeless Hair

You may have beautiful, fragile hair, but it is lifeless. This condition will lead to the hair breaking easily, especially when they are dry and have split ends. This hair will have limpness in nature and lack bounce. The causes of weak hair may be genetic and can be worsened by chemical treatments, heat damage, environmental factors, and pressure from having the same hairstyle.

Oily and Greasy Hair

Human skin is full of pores joined to sebaceous

glands that reveal a natural oil known as sebum. It is the function of sebum to keep hair soft, manageable, and smooth.

Though sebum is expected to keep the hair soft and smooth, the scalp produces excess sebum that leads to oily and greasy hair. Factors that cause oily and greasy hair may be natural causes that include hair type, hormones, genetics, and skin condition like psoriasis, eczema, and seborrheic dermatitis.

Other causes that are human made are frequent brushing of hair, frequent shampooing and conditioning of hair, or tying your hair too tight. Another cause that we are not serious about is the regular use of hot water on the hair. Hot water stimulates the sebaceous glands and makes them produce more sebum.

Dandruff

Dandruff is a condition where the skin of the scalp is peeling off and flakes. Most times, people thought that this symptom is a sign of poor hygiene, but many reasons contribute to dandruff.

Among other reasons, seborrheic dermatitis can be a cause of severe dandruff. This is a situation when the skin is overactive, thereby leading to the scalp been irritated and produces extra skin cells. The moment the skin cell die, they will fall off and form what is known as dandruff. Other factors that lead to dandruff are known as psoriasis and eczema. Another condition that can lead to dandruff is when the skin is too dry, especially during winter. Also, some hair care products can cause dandruff. Such products will trigger a red, itchy scalp.

Sensitive Scalps

When the scalp is sensitive, it will be feeling itchy and irritated. When a scalp is sensitive, it will bring out some conditions such as tightness, itchiness, and there will be pain at the root. The imbalance of sebum secretion that leads to irritation can be one of the sources of scalp sensitivity. Pollution that coat hair can also be one of the causes as it will create a dull film on the hair and create free radicals.

Stress can also be one of the significant factors that will determine the condition of hair and scalp. Other reasons include the use of harsh hair care products, improper diet, sun rays, chlorinated water, blow-drying and frequent styling.

Color and Bleach Damaged Hair

Harsh chemicals are exposed to hair when you dye it. These harsh chemicals can damage the hair. Whenever the hair is exposed to harsh chemicals, the follicles become very porous and filled with small holes due to color, and hair protein gotten from the hair has to be used for the hair to be brightened.

Bleaching of hair makes it raise its outer cuticle for the bleaching agents to penetrate. Whereas repeated bleaching of the hair will build the cuticle scale, thereby allowing it to lose moisture. Bleaching will lead to hair been broken and having split ends.

Dry Hair

When hair is finding it challenging to retain the moisture, it will lead to dry hair. Dry hair is a condition where the hair will be less shiny, appearing dull and lifeless. It is a sign of unhealthy hair, and those different kinds of factors that include environmental conditions, hair conditions, and exposure to harsh hair products are part of what may have caused it.

Dry climates, frequently swimming in salty or chlorinated water, too much exposure to wind or sun, is part of the environmental factors that affect hair. Others are exposure to harsh chemicals, frequent washing of hair, dyeing of hair, and frequent use of blow dryers, straighteners, and curling irons.

Frizzy Hair

This is a result of a raised cuticle that allows moisture to enter the hair and swell the strand. Frizzy hair will get worse in either rainy days or humidity, as the hair will absorb added moisture. The cause of Frizzy hair includes dehydration of hair. Hair throughout the day will absorb moisture from the atmosphere for the cuticle to open up.

Heat Damaged Hair

Straight, wavy or curly hair will require styling with hot tools to get the desired results. Though hot styling tools are fantastic ways to make us look amazing, the problems come when they are overused or are incorrectly used. Heat damaged may happen in one simple curls or swipe or when overexposed to them.

Hair Loss

Hair loss causes low self-esteem. Hair loss can be a result of genetic and hormonal factors. Hair loss happens when the androgen hormones in the body that shrinks hair follicle is not growing again. Genetic is not the only reason for hair loss, and it may be due to alopecia areata, an autoimmune situation where an immune system attack hair follicles.

It may also be a result of hormonal imbalances that occur during pregnancy. Hair loss can sometimes be a result of medications and medical treatments and sicknesses. Another factor is when the body has gone through sudden shock or stress, which will lead to hair loss.

Split Ends

This situation occurs when the hair shaft frays or split because of some reason. Damage to the hair will show at the end of the hair and can also be seen anywhere on the hair. The causes of split ends are stress form factors like environmental, mechanical, and physical. Another set of factors that can also cause split ends is excessive blow-drying, frequent brushing, and hair strength. Other significant factors are diet and hormones.

Grey Hair

Grey hair is a natural indication of old age, and there is nothing wrong with having it when aging. Grey hair occurs naturally when cells known as melanin are not producing again. The rate of growing grey depends on genetics. Also stress, hormonal and nutritional factors can affect the color of the hair.

HAIR AND SCALP TREATMENTS

This is not rocket science. You can have shiny, healthy hair if you eat a healthy diet. Balanced food nourishes the entire body, including scalp and hair.

Whenever you want to buy hair care products, avoid those that are chemical-based. If you discovered that the shampoo you are using is causing your hair problems, leave it for another type or brand. Remember that the popularity of a brand is not a sure way of having shiny hair.

There are many natural-based ingredients hair care products in the market, like herbal hair oil-infused products. Though some of them are expensive, the result cannot be over-emphasized. But if you decide to go natural such as herbal oils infused or herbal rinsed, this book is sure to guide you.

Chapter 2

HERBAL HAIR OIL INFUSION

Prolong usage of harsh chemical-based hair products will damage hair seriously. If you want to make your hair shiny and beautiful, natural ingredients are readily available, although they cost, and the prices depend on the brand.

This guide is all about everything you want to know about natural herbs. It will familiarize you with the essential elements of herbal oil infusion that include common herbs that will bring about healthy and shiny hair.

Herbs are parts of plants or plants that are useful for medicinal, aromatic, and savory characteristics.

Ways to Prepare Herbs

We have many ways to prepare herbs as at today. The preparation of herbs depends on the ways you want to use the end products.

Oil infusion: This method is achieved by the combination of crushed herbs and oil. Preferably the crushed herbs should be dry. The mixture of herbs and oil and can be done either under the sun or making use of a double boiler.

Tinctures: Tinctures can be gotten when water and alcohol solution is used to soak the herbs. The alcohol will act to preserve the active ingredients of the herb. The Extracted solution form the mixture will be stored in a sterilized bottle. The tincture should be mixed with water before drinking.

Creams: When preparing creams, herbs and oils have to be simmering for three hours. The liquid from the simmering will be stored in a sterilized dark bottle.

Decoctions: This is a mixture of berries, barks, and roots in boiled water to extract the active ingredients. The concoction will now be strained and stored in sterilized water. This decoction can be taken hot or cold like water.

Ointments: To achieve this method, heat both oil or fat and herb quickly in a boiler. Then strained and allowing solidified.

Drink infusion: You can achieve this solution

by boiling herbs with water to create tea.

WHAT IS AN HERBAL HAIR OIL INFUSION

Herbal hair oil is the outcome of the mixture of herbs and oil or fat. It does not matter whether the type of herb, either dry or fresh, will give the herbal hair infusion. Though there is a recommendation that to achieve the desired outcome, it is better to make use of the dried herbs as it helps in avoiding the bacterial that may be coming from the natural moisture of the fresh herbs

If you want to escape the stress of straining the infused oil, it is recommended to use essential oils though expensive. Note that infusion is achieved by heating oil or fat and herb with either cooking or solar method.

Cooking Method: With this method, you heat the mixture in a double boiler making use of low fire until the infusion is achieved. This method is efficient and quicker.

Solar Method: With this method, the heating will be done under the sun. The solar process is tedious and consumes time, as it will take a longer time to achieve infusion.

Basic components of herbal hair infusion;

Dried herbs or essential oils.

Carrier oils.

HOW TO PREPARE HERBAL OIL INFUSION

Observe the following when you want to make a basic herbal hair oil infusion;

Container: Select and use a clean and dry container for infused oil. The bottle to be used should be sterilized and allow to dry. The recommended container should those with cork lids and not metal lids to avoid been rusty.

Herbs: Select herbs that will give you the desired end products. Don't forget, as mentioned earlier, that dried herbs are better than the fresh herbs. Note that bacterial grow faster in fresh herbs due to its natural moisture.

Carrier oil: Several kinds of research have shown that Jojoba and Olive oil have the most extended shelf life among the carrier oils. Almond has been discovered to be the most used as it gives sweet fragrant aroma.

Note that infusion is achieved by sun heat method, cold method, and heating method.

COMMON HERBS FOR THE TREATMENT OF HAIR AND SCALP

We have many herbs, but remember that not all herbs have the needed properties to care for your hair and scalp. Herbs are known to be associated with cooking when a flavor is required to be added to food, though some herbs present more benefits like taking care of hair and scalp.

There are many herbs at the supermarket, but the following are some of the most common to find for the treatment of hair and scalp.

Herb	Source	Benefits
Rosemary	Mediterranean	• Helps in nourishes dry scalp • Aids growth of hair • Reduce early graying • Prevents dandruff
Lavender	Mediterranean, India, Middle East	• Aids hair growth • Helps in soothing scalp infections
Aloe Vera	North Africa	• Possess Aloenin that helps in the regeneration of hair cells • Acts as a conditioner for hair • Aids the growth and thickness of hair
Lemongrass	Sri Lanka, India, Thailand, Burma	• Helps in strengthening of hair • Assists in the prevention of hair loss

		• Controls scalp inflammation
Sage	Mediterranean	• Prevents dandruff • Used for the treatment of scalp infections • Brings back hair color • Great for oily hair
Basil	India	• Helps in the removal of flakes • Controls dandruff
Chamomile	Ancient Egypt, Rome	• Helps in soothing the scalp • Good conditioner and helps in soften hair • Used to strengthening the scalp • Helps in adding shine to blond and fair hair
Yucca Root	Mexico, North America	• Used for the prevention of hair loss • Treats Dandruff

		• Used to soothe and nourishes the scalp • Acts as a natural cleansing and foaming
Henna	India, Ancient Egypt	• Can be used to seal moisture in the hair • Acts as a natural dye • Good deep conditioners for hair
Burdock	Europe, Northern Asia	• Used for the prevention of hair loss • Enhances hair body and luster • Used to smoothens tangles

Chapter 3

CARRIER OILS

In making herbal hair infusion, carrier oil is one of the essential ingredients. That is the main reason this chapter is dedicated to carrier oils, properties, extractions, and uses. Not forgetting to discuss some common carrier oils that help in the treatment and management of hair and scalp.

ABOUT CARRIER OILS

Carrier oils are known to be vegetable or base oils that are gotten from seeds, nuts, or other fatty plant or its parts. Carrier oils go into unpleasant smell over time, and their aroma is not as sharp as that of essential oils.

Some carrier oils are gotten from animal fossils, but they are not suitable for personal care and aromatherapy infusions. We discovered that some beauty products and personal care products contain mineral oil, but they are not suitable carrier oils.

ESSENTIAL FATTY ACIDS

The human body naturally generates fatty acids to maintain warmness and healthy. Those that cannot produce naturally by the human body are gotten through the consumption of balanced food. Among the functions of fatty acids is to keep the body healthy and help maintain the skin's natural moisture. The essential fatty acids for the human body are Linoleic Acid and Alpha-Linoleic Acid.

USES OF CARRIER OIL

The primary objective of carrier oil is to act as a diffuser or carrying agent for essential oil. Since essential oil will cause irritation in its purest form, it is why carrier oil is added. The carrier oil will dilute the intense potency of the essential oil.

PREPARATION OF CARRIER OIL

There are three ways to prepare carrier oil;

By solvent extraction: With this method, the solvent will be used to extract the carrier oil. The disadvantage of this method is that it will destroy the oil's fatty acids and natural nutrients, thereby leaving only the remnant of the solvent that is mixed with the oil.

By cold pressing: Preparation by cold pressing is the most common method. In this method, the oil is extracted from the fatty portion of the botanical plant. When using the pressing machine, there will be natural heat gotten from the friction of the machine.

By cold expeller pressed: This is very similar to the cold pressing method of preparing carrier oil. But the difference is that the extra heat is kept to a minimum because the cold condition of the machine is needed to be able to keep the natural nutrients in the oil.

PROPERTIES OF CARRIER OIL

After the carrier oil has been extracted, its feature will change from a virgin, extra virgin, refined, and unrefined.

Virgin or extra virgin oil: This form applies to

Olive oil. The extra virgin is gotten by cold pressing the olives once. If you want more from the olives, you extract more with the aid of the cold press to extract virgin oil.

Refined or Fractionated oil: This form of oil is gotten to improve the shelf life of the oil. The disadvantage of this is that it will destroy the nutrients, vitamins, and fatty acids in the oil.

Unrefined oil: This is achieved when the carrier oil is filtered to get rid of small particles and dust without affecting the natural condition of its fatty acids, nutrients, and vitamins.

Note: The oil with the best quality is the unrefined oil.

COMMON CARRIERS OILS AND BENEFITS

Some many seeds and plants are sources of abundant fatty acids and can be used as carrier oils, but we have discovered that not all of them can be used to treat hair and scalp.

It is essential to be aware that the oil's absorption rate will determine the type of oil that will best suit your skin, hair, and scalp. It has been discovered that fast absorption oils are for oily skin, the average absorption is for the normal skin, and the slow absorption is for those with dry and mature skin.

The table below shows common carrier oils used in the preparation of your herbal hair infusion.

Carrier Oil	Source	Benefits	Absorption
Coconut oil	Asia, Africa, Polynesia	• Great for dry hair • Enhances splits ends	Slow
Jojoba oil	Southern California, Southern Arizona, Northwestern	• Helps in the dissolution of Sebum • Enhances	Average

	Mexico	dry scalp	
Olive oil	Greece, Mediterranean	• Great for dry hair • Aids hair shiny and healthy • Controls dandruff	Slow
Apricot oil	Armenia	• Great for oily hair and scalp • Use to prevent loss of hair • Controls scalp moisture • Enhances hair growth	Fast
Sweet Almond oil	Central Asia, China	• Great for hair • Helps in the nourishment and	Slow

		strengthening of hair • Aids the treatments of hair damage	
Argan oil	Morocco	• Great for normal hair • Acts as a conditioner for hair • Makes hair soft and shiny • Prevent frizzy hair • Help in the treatments of split ends	Average
Avocado oil	South Central Mexico	• Great for dry hair • Enhances blood flow in the scalp	Slow
Sesame	India, Africa	• Helps in the strengthening	Average

oil		of hair from roots to the tips • Controls premature graying • Prevent dandruff • Good for dry hair	
Hazel oil	Rome	• Helps in the growth of hair • Enhances hair and scalp • Assists in the stimulation of hair follicles	Fast
Grape seed Oil	North America	• Aids the growth of hair • Good for	Fast

| | | oily hair

• Keeps scalp healthy

• Makes hair shiny and non-greasy | |

Chapter 4

USES OF ESSENTIAL OILS

The general notion is that essential oils originated from Ancient Egypt. History made us know that since time immemorial, Egyptians have been using oils for beauty and embalming purposes. So this chapter covers all about essential oils, its preparation, uses, and its benefits. Other discussions will include how to use essential oils with carrier oils, and a guide on how to convert natural essential oil for hair and the treatment of scalp.

WHAT ARE ESSENTIAL OILS

Essential oils are extracted from flowers, barks, roots, leave, and other parts of a plant.

Uses of Essential Oils

Essential oils have become essential needs as they can be used for different purposes. Most of the common essential oils possess aromatherapy properties, healing properties, soothing and aesthetic characteristics. All these properties can either be in their purest form or mixed with other types of oils.

Uses of Essential oils for the treatment of hair;

1. Hair shampoo.

2. Treatment of dandruff.

3. Acts as a hair conditioner.

4. Treatment of itchy scalp.

5. Makes hair thicker.

6. Suitable for dry hair.

Other uses of essential oils are;

At home:

1. Acts as a deodorizer.

2. They are used as an all-purpose cleaner.

3. Food coloring.

4. Acts as a mosquito repellant.

For Medicinal:

1. for burns.

2. for indigestion.

3. To treat headaches.

4. for the treatment of coughs and sinusitis.

5. for relaxation and Spa:

6. for Sauna/Massage.

7. for Detox.

8. To improve sleep.

THE EXTRACTION OF ESSENTIAL OIL

Pure essential oil is extracted with any of the following methods, according to the National Association of Holistic Aromatherapy (NAHA).

• Distillation

• Effleurage

• Cold Pressing or Expression

• CO$_2$ Extraction

• Solvent Extraction

Among the above processes, distillation and Expression are the standard methods of extracting pure essential oils. Though some

people prefer infusion as a way to obtain the essential oil, the disadvantage is that the infusion of herb with carrier oil will only dilute the essential oil as it will not consider as a pure essential oil.

Distillation is a method of separating the plant's organic compound with the aid of water through condensation and vaporization. There are three types of distillation and are; steam distillation, water distillation, and the combination of steam and water distillation.

However, the Expression, also known as cold pressing, is applied particularly on citrus plants that include lemon, oranges, lime, bergamot, and tangerine. The standard method of extracting essential oils in ancient times is cold pressing, an old-fashioned way of making use of a sponge to extract the essential oil.

With the technology, cold pressing is achieved with a method known as ecuelle a piquer. This method involves making use of a container with spikes to prick and prod the seeds until the essential oil is extracted.

DANGERS OF ESSENTIAL OILS

There have several recommendations that essential oils are some of the best alternatives for most health care remedies due to their organic components.

However, the use of essential oils has its disadvantages. Improper use of essential oil may lead to several dangerous effects.

1. Remember that some oils can cause burning and discoloration as they have reactions when exposed to sunlight. Some of these can cause allergy or skin issues. Note that cumin oils and citrus oils are photosensitive oils.

2. Essential oils, such as lemongrass oils and peppermint oils, when applied to the skin undiluted, may lead to itching and irritation.

3. Wintergreen and sage oils can lead to adverse effects on babies and pregnant even when diluted.

4. Don't inhale essential oils directly as it will portray potential dangers to breathing.

5. Not all essential oils are suitable for pets.

6. Consult your doctor before you decide to drink essential oils even if diluted, as it may lead to death to those that are allergic to it.

CONVERSION OF ESSENTIAL OILS

The table below is the standard unit of conversion and dilution for essential oil. This table will help when you want to prepare the herbal oil infusion recipe.

Milliliters (ml)	Ounces (oz.)	Drops
1	0.033	20
3.75	1/8	75
5	1/6	100

7.5	1/4	150
10	1/3	200
15	1/2	300
30	1	600
60	2	1200
120	4	2400
180	6	3600
249	8	4800

It is recommended that essential oil should not be more than 1-2% of the total finished mixture.

If the dilution is 1%, add 12 drops of your essential oil to a 60 ml bottle of lotion.

60 ml = 1200 drops

1% of 1200 drops = 12 drops

ESSENTIAL OILS FOR HAIR AND SCALP TREATMENT

There are many plants that can be used to extract essential oils, but not all are for the treatment of hair and scalp. The most common are those listed in chapter 2, and they can be combined to have your recipe.

In the table below are the useful essential oils that are needed for your hair and the treatment of scalp.

Essential Oil	Source	Benefits to Hair
Rosemary	Mediterranean	• Makes hair and scalp healthier • Suitable for the prevention of hair loss • Enhances hair growth

		• Strengthening hair
		• Useful for the treatment of alopecia areata
Lavender	India, Mediterranean	• Excellent antiseptic and anti-inflammatory properties
		• Helps in the treatment of scalp inflammation
		• Controls dandruff
		• Helps in reduction of hair loss
		makes hair shines
		• Helps to nourishes and soothe irritation against flaky skin and dry hair
Chamomile	Ancient Egypt, Rome	• Guard against scalp inflammation
		• Suitable for the prevention of hair

		loss
		• Great for the treatment of itchy scalp
Ylang Ylang	Philippines	• Improve the thickness of hair • Suitable for the reduction of split ends • Suitable for the improvement of oil balance in the scalp • Makes hair healthier and fuller

Chapter 5

DIY (DO-IT-YOURSELF) PROCEDURES FOR HAIR TREATMENT

This chapter will be for how to DIY recipes for regular hair oil infusion for the treatment of hair. There are many ways to take care of your hair. And that is what this chapter is intended to do and also to portray the benefits of each recipe.

HOT OIL TREATMENT

Hot oil treatment is widely used for the prevention of hair been damaged or to safeguard the damage of hair. Hot oil is applied gently on the scalp to cover the roots and tips of the hair.

Benefits of Hot Oil Treatment

1. Hot oil treatment will act as a conditioner on the hair, giving it a shiny and vibrant color.

2. Hot oil treatment will help in the treatment of hair damaged by the sun and harsh chemicals based products.

3. It will help to increase the circulation of blood on the scalp.

4. They will moisture brittle and dry hair.

Note that hot oil treatment should be prepared once a week if the hair to be treated is dry and brittle. Massage the hair with hot oil and leave it for 30 minutes or more depending on the damaged hair level.

HOT OIL TREATMENT RECIPES

YLANG COCONUT HOT OIL TREATMENT (NORMAL HAIR)

Ingredients:

8 oz. Coconut oil

48 Drops Ylang Ylang

Methods:

1. Pour water into a saucepan and boil on high heat.

2. Lower the heat to low to keep the water simmering.

3. Make use of 1% dilution, measure 48 drops of Ylang Ylang essential oil.

4. Combine Ylang Ylang and coconut in a heatproof container.

5. Transfer the container to the simmering water to infuse the oil.

6. Allow the infuse oil cooling.

7. Keep it in an amber-colored container.

Application:

• Pour six tablespoons of the oil into a container.

• Place the container in boiled water. Allow feeling warm when touched.

• Pour the heated oil into the scalp.

• Massage the oil slowly on the scalp to the tip of the hair until well coated.

• Cover the head with a shower cap and allow resting for 30 minutes or overnight.

• Shampoo and rinse after resting thoroughly to remove excess oil.

Storage: Keep the remaining oil in an amber-colored jar in a dry, cool place.

Shelf life: 1 to 2 years

OLIVE-AVOCADO HOT OIL TREATMENT

Ingredients:

4 Tablespoons of Avocado oil

4 Tablespoons of Olive oil

4 Tablespoons of Jojoba oil

2 Bunches of Rosemary (fresh)

12-15 drops Peppermint essential oil

Methods:

1. Pour water into a saucepan and place on high heat to boil.

2. Lower the heat to low and allow the water to simmering.

3. Combine avocado oil, olive oil, jojoba oil in a heatproof container.

4. Add in the fresh rosemary and mix well (must be dry and has no moisture).

5. Transfer the heatproof container into the simmering water.

6. Allow infusing for 45 minutes.

7. Check always to avoid been dried up.

8. After infused, allow to cool a bit, but it must be warm, and then add peppermint essential oil.

9. Pour the infused oil into an airtight container.

Application:

• Pour a quarter of the mixture into a container.

• Use your fingers to apply it to the scalp.

• Massage the oil gently from your scalp to the tip.

•Massage until well coated.

• Cover the head with a shower cap.

• Shampoo and rinse after resting thoroughly to

remove excess oil.

• Repeat the process every 2 to 4 weeks to be able to have better results.

Storage: Store the mixture in a heatproof and airtight container.

• Allow it cool before closing the cover.

• Store in a dark place.

Shelf life: Shelf life is 2 to 4 weeks. Don't use fresh herbs so as not to shorten the shelf life.

ARGAN-JOJOBA HOT OIL TREATMENT (FRIZZY HAIR)

Ingredients:

4 Tablespoons of Argan oil

4 Tablespoons of Jojoba Oil

12 Drops of Burdock oil

Methods:

1. Pour water in a saucepan and place on high heat.

2. Lower the heat to low and allow the water to simmering.

3. Combine argan oil, jojoba oil, and burdock in a heatproof container.

4. Transfer the container to the simmering water to infuse the oil.

5. Allow the infused oil cool.

6. Pour the oil in an amber-colored jar.

Application:

• Pour a quarter of the infused oil in a

container.

• Place the container in boiled water. Do not allow boiling; just allow feeling warm.

• Apply the warm oil to the scalp.

• Massage the oil slowly from the scalp to the tip of the hair until well coated.

• Cover your head with a shower cap and allow resting for 30 minutes or overnight.

• Shampoo and rinse after resting thoroughly to remove excess oil.

Storage: Store in an amber-colored jar and keep in a dry, cool place.

Shelf life: 1 to 2 years if stored correctly.

Deep conditioner treatment is a way to restore the strength and health of hair. This method makes hair to withstand the stress of everyday styling and constant coloring of hair.

Benefits of Deep Conditioner Treatment

1. Deep conditioner treatment helps in protecting the hair from possible damages such as split ends, brittleness, drying, and breakages.

2. It helps to retain the natural moisture of hair to keep it healthy and strong.

3. Adding the treatment to your hair will soften it and leave it silky and shiny.

Note that deep conditioner treatment should be applied one to two times if there is damaged or dry hair.

Deep Conditioner Treatment Recipes

Coconut Oil Deep Conditioner

Ingredients:

2 Tablespoons of Jojoba oil

4 Tablespoons of Coconut oil

6 Drops of Lavender essential oil

Methods:

1. Place the coconut oil for a few minutes in a fridge to solidify.

2. Pour the coconut into a bowl and melts until

it turns creamy.

3. Add jojoba oil and blend until well blended.

4. Then add lavender essential oil.

5. Mix until the mixture is well blended.

Application:

• Use your finger to scoop up the creamy oil from the bowl.

• Massage gently with your finger on the scalp.

• Apply from the roots to the tip of the hair.

• Apply until the hair is well coated.

• Cover the head with a shower cap.

• Use a hairdryer to heat the treatment or put a warm towel under the shower cap.

• Allow the treatment on the hair for 25 minutes.

• Repeat the process once a week.

Storage: keep the leftover in the fridge to keep the coconut oil in a solid-state.

Shelf life: The mixture should be for two-time usage.

OLIVE-YLANG YLANG OIL DEEP CONDITIONER

Ingredients:

2 Tablespoons of Olive oil

6 Tablespoons of Coconut oil

16 Drops of Ylang Ylang essential oil

Hand mixer

Methods:

1. Mix olive oil, coconut oil, and essential oil in a bowl.

2. Use the hand mixer to mix the mixture until it becomes thick and creamy.

Application:

• Scoop up the whipped mix into clean, dry hair.

• Use comb to spread it well on the hair.

• Allow it to rest for 20 minutes.

• Wash and shampoo it.

• Repeat the method once a week or as you wish.

Storage: Not to be stored under the sun.

Shelf life: Not to be stored as it turns into

foam.

**SHEA AND COCONUT DEEP
CONDITIONER**

Ingredients:

2 Tablespoons of Shea butter

4 Tablespoons of Coconut oil

2 Teaspoons of Argan oil

6 drops of Rosemary essential oil

Methods:

1. Pour both the coconut oil and Shea butter into a bowl in a solid form.

2. Transfer to the microwave to melt.

3. Allow cool to become creamy.

4. Then add argan oil and rosemary essential oil.

5. Whip the mixture for 5 minutes or until it turns creamy.

Application:

• Massage to the hair.

• Use a comb to spread the mixture evenly

• Allow resting for 30 minutes.

• Shampoo and Wash it thoroughly.

Storage: Prepare one application.

Shelf life: Not to be stored.

Pre-poo Hair Oil Treatment and Recipes

It is evident that whenever shampoo is applied to hair, it will leave some residues that make hair dull and heavy. Harsh properties in commercial shampoo may take away the shine and luster of hair. This condition is the reason why a treatment called pre-poo is needed.

Pre-poo, also known as Pre-shampoo, is a kind of treatment for hair care. This treatment is done to prevent stripping hair of its natural moisture and oils due to frequent shampooing.

Benefits of Pre-poo hair oil treatment

1. This treatment will restore hair's moisture.

2. Helps in the restoration of shining hair.

3. Protects hair from the shampoo harsh effects.

4. It aids the softening of the hair.

<h2 style="text-align:center">PRE-POO HAIR OIL TREATMENT RECIPES</h2>

<h3 style="text-align:center">VIRGIN OLIVE PRE-POO HAIR TREATMENT</h3>

Ingredients:

4 Tablespoons of Virgin Olive oil

5 drops of Tea tree essential oil

2 Tablespoons of Castor oil

Methods:

1. Mix tea tree essential oil with olive oil and castor oil in a spritzer.

2. Blend the mixture until well mixed.

Application:

• Spray the mixture from the roots of the hair to the tip.

• Cover the hair with plastic or shower cap for 20 minutes or more.

• Remove the cap and massage the scalp.

• Wash and shampoo the hair.

• Do this once or twice a week.

Storage: Keep the leftover in the spritzer bottle for easy use.

Shelf life: Not more than two-time applications.

Coco-Avocado Mask

Ingredients:

1 ripe Avocado (small)

1 Tablespoon of Coconut oil

1 Tablespoon of Olive oil

1 Tablespoon of Castor oil

Methods:

1. Mash the avocado until it turns thick and creamy.

2. Then add castor oil, coconut oil, and olive oil.

3. Blend the mixture until well blended.

Application:

• Apply the mixture into the hair from the roots

to the tip.

• Leave the mixture on the hair overnight.

• Cover the hair with a plastic cap or shower cap.

• Shampoo and wash the hair well to remove the avocado residue.

Storage: Avocado will tend to spoil, so it is better to prepare for one usage.

Shelf life: Not more than one application.

ALMOND-OLIVE PRE-POO

Ingredients:

4 Tablespoons of Olive oil

4 Tablespoons of Almond oil

4 Tablespoons of Castor oil

Methods:

1. Combine the entire ingredients in a spritzer bottle.

2. Shake the mixture thoroughly.

Application:

• Spray the mixture starting from the roots to the tip of the hair.

• Cover the hair with a shower cap for 20 minutes or more.

• Remove the cap and massage the scalp well.

• Shampoo and rinse the hair thoroughly.

• Do this treatment once a week.

Storage: Keep the mixture in the spritzer bottle.

Shelf life: Not more than two-time applications.

LEAVE-IN HAIR OIL TREATMENT AND RECIPES

Leave-in Hair Oil Treatment is performed on hair to control frizzy hairs.

Benefits Leave-in Hair Oil Treatment

A good leave-in conditioner will be of advantage in these ways;

1. Controls the flying away of hair.

2. It helps to manage frizzy hair.

3. Help in detangling of hair.

Note that the Leave-in conditioner is applied after shampoo to be able to manage the harm curls. So it can be used as often as possible.

LEAVE-IN HAIR CONDITIONER RECIPES

ALOE VERA DETANGLER LEAVE IN CONDITIONER

Ingredients:

3/4 Cup Distilled water

2 Tablespoons Aloe Vera gel

20 drops Rosemary essential oil

2 Tablespoons Vegetable glycerin

Methods:

1. Pour the Aloe Vera gel in a spray bottle.

2. Add distilled water.

3. Pour in vegetable glycerin.

4. Stir in rosemary essential oil.

5. Cover the spray bottle and shake until well blended.

Application:

• Wet your hair.

• Spray the conditioner to detangle the hair.

• Use brush to get rid of tangles.

Storage: Keep the conditioner in a spritzer bottle.

Shelf life: Due to water content, bacteria may set in. So don't have more leftovers.

Aloe Vera-Coconut Leave-in Conditioner

Ingredients:

4 oz. Aloe Vera gel

2 oz. Coconut oil

2 Teaspoons of Avocado oil

Methods:

1. Mix the entire ingredients in a bowl.

2. Use a mixer to blend the mixture until it turns thick and creamy.

Application:

• Wet your hair.

• Apply the mixture to the hair.

• Comb the hair until the mixture is spread everywhere on the hair.

Storage: Store in a cool, dry place.

Shelf life: Not more than two-time applications.

Chapter 6

HERBAL OIL INFUSION RECIPE FOR SCALP TREATMENT

A healthy scalp makes healthy hair.

This chapter is about some do it yourself recipes that will help in the treatment of your scalp and the removal of dandruff.

DRY SCALP TREATMENT

When the scalp is dry, it will affect the growth and health of hair. To have healthy hair, it is essential to treat the scalp as much as the hair is treated. So scalp treatment is a way of treating scalp to nourish the scalp with the use of massage oils. Serious cases of the dry scalp will lead to skin inflammation that shows symptoms such as itchiness, redness, and flakiness.

Benefits of Treating Scalp with oil treatment

Other major health problems associated with severe dry scalp are flakiness and dandruff. Most times, what causes these health problems are the advice effects of chemical-based hair care products at the supermarkets. So it is advisable to use naturally based treatments like Olive oil to care for your scalp.

Note that the scalp needed to be treated at least two times a week.

Below are some of such oil treatment recipes

for dry scalp:

DRY SCALP TREATMENT RECIPES

TREE TEA-OLIVE OIL TREATMENT

Ingredients:

4 drops Tea tree essential oil

2 oz. Extra Virgin Olive oil

Methods:

1. Combine both the tea tree and olive in a container.

2. Shake the mixture very well.

Application:

• Apply the mixture to the dry scalp.

• Massage the scalp very well.

• Comb the hair gently to remove flakes.

• Leave the scalp for 30 minutes or more.

• Shampoo and rinse the hair.

• Do these procedures again after two days.

Storage: Store in a dry, cool place.

Shelf life: Not more than two-time applications.

PEPPERMINT OIL TREATMENT

Ingredients:

4 drops Peppermint essential oil

2 oz. Coconut oil

Methods:

1. Dilute the peppermint essential oil with coconut in a container.

2. Shake the mixture in the container until well mixed.

Application:

• Apply the mixture directly into the scalp.

• Massage the scalp very well.

• Comb the hair gently to remove flakes.

• Leave the scalp for 30 minutes or more.

• Shampoo and rinse the hair.

• Do these procedures again after two days.

Storage: Store in a dry, cool place.

Shelf life: Not more than two-time applications.

Avocado Paste oil treatment

Ingredients:

1 ripe Avocado (small)

1 Teaspoon Honey (organic)

2 Tablespoons Olive oil

Methods:

1. Mash the avocado in a bowl until it turns to paste.

2. Add honey and olive oil.

3. Blend the mixture until well combined.

Application:

• Apply the avocado paste to the scalp.

• Massage the scalp gently.

• Leave the scalp for 30 minutes or more.

• Shampoo and rinse the hair.

Storage: Not more than once, as the avocado will tend to spoil.

Shelf life: One application.

ITCHY SCALP TREATMENT

Itchy scalp is known to be caused by a dry scalp and can lead to dandruff.

Benefits of treating itchy scalp

1. Ability to remove itchiness and redness.

2. Ability to avoid early hair loss.

3. Ability to prevent dandruff.

Note that the recipes recommended can be used for the treatment of itchy scalp two times a week.

ITCHY SCALP TREATMENT RECIPES

TEA TREE-OLIVE OIL

Ingredients:

6 drops Tea tree essential oil

2 Tablespoons Olive oil

Methods:

1. Combine tree tea oil and olive oil in a container.

Application:

• Apply the mixture to the scalp and spread evenly to the hair.

• Allow rest on the hair for 30 minutes or more.

• Brush the hair in other to remove flakes.

• Shampoo and rinse the hair well.

• Do these procedures 2-3 times per week.

Storage: keep in a dry, cool place

Shelf life: Not more than two applications.

HOMEMADE ESSENTIAL OILS FOR ITCHY SCALP

Ingredients:

2 cup virgin coconut oil

5 sprigs Rosemary essential leaves (fresh)

12 drops Rosemary essential oil

12 drops Lavender essential oil

10 drops Patchouli essential oil

12 drops Tea tree essential oil

2 Cups Water

1 Cup Apple cider vinegar

Methods:

1. Dilute the raw apple cider with the water.

2. Wash and towel dry the rosemary to avoid water moisture that may make the oil rancid.

3. Combine rosemary leave and coconut oil in a double boiler.

4. Allow the mixture for 3 hours to infuse on low heat.

5. Simmer the mixture and stir.

6. Pour the infused oil into a container, and then strain the liquid.

7. Allow cooling for 5 minutes.

8. Add all the essential oils and stir.

Application:

• Scoop up the infused oil with fingers.

• Apply the mix to the roots and scalp, making sure it spread evenly.

• Cover the hair with a shower cap for 50-60 minutes.

• Wash the hair with clear water to get rid of oil.

•Shampoo and condition the hair after washing.

• Apply the diluted apple cider on the scalp.

• Massage the scalp and rinse the hair well.

• Do these procedures 2-3 times per week.

Storage: Store in a cool, dry place.

Shelf life: Not more than two applications.

Chapter 7

HERBAL OIL INFUSION RECIPE FOR REGULAR HAIR TREATMENT

As discussed earlier, most hair problems are caused by harsh chemicals in commercial hair care products, genetic, environment, prolong exposure to sunlight, and improper care.

This chapter will cover the most common hair problems that may occur and the corresponding homemade recipes treatments to get rid of them.

Dry/Heat Damaged Hair Treatment

Dry hair is known to be dull, lifeless stands and frizzy hair. Dry hair is caused by a lack of moisture in the hair. Dry hair will lead to damaged hair, such as split ends and brittleness.

Don't forget that shampoo residue, as discussed earlier, will make hair dry and heavy. Also, constant styling and drying of hair will make your hair dry and be damaged.

Dry Hair Treatment

The essence of dry hair treatment is to give hair back life and nourishment, as hair needs moisture to be strong and healthy. If dry hair is left untreated, it will lead to other hair issues that may include loss of hair.

Benefits of Treating Dry Hair

1. Giving hair vibrancy.

2. Hair will be healthy and strong.

3. Ability to manage your hair better.

Note that treating dry hair should be a weekly procedure for the hair to have regular nourishment.

DRY/HEAT DAMAGED HAIR TREATMENT RECIPES

COCO-VERA CONDITIONER

Ingredients:

1 Cup Coconut oil

2 Aloe Vera leaves

10 drops rosemary essential oil

Methods:

1. Take a knife to cut the Aloe Vera leaves into pieces.

2. Scrap the Aloe Vera gel and pour it into a bowl.

3. Then add coconut oil.

4. Place the mixture on low heat for 10-15 minutes.

5. Allow the mixture to cool completely.

6. Add the rosemary essential oil.

7. Mix the ingredients and pour into a container and close the lid.

Application:

• Take the desired portion into a jar and warm it slightly.

• Apply the mixture from the roots to the tip of the hair.

• Massage the oil for some minutes into the scalp to enhance the blood circulation.

• Rinse the hair and apply mild shampoo and conditioner.

•Do the procedure two times per week.

Storage: Store in a cool place.

Shelf life: Not more than two weeks.

Ingredients:

4 cloves of Garlic

1 red Onion

3/4 cup Coconut oil

8 drops Lavender essential oil

2 Teaspoons Lemon juice

Water

Methods:

1. Mix chopped garlic, onion, and coconut oil in a pan.

2. Place the mixture on low flame and heat until it stops bubbling.

3. Allow cooling completely.

4. Add lavender essential oil.

5. Pour the mixture in a bowl, strain, and into a bottle.

6. In another bowl, combine lemon juice with water for dilution.

Application:

•Massage the oil mix into the scalp.

• Cover the head with a hot towel.

• Allow the oil to soak the hair for up to 20 minutes.

• Rinse, shampoo and apply conditioner to the hair.

• Use the diluted lemon juice as a rinse to remove the smell of the non-garlic mixture.

Storage: Store in a container and place it in a fridge.

Shelf life: Not more than ten days.

AVOCADO OIL FOR HEAT DAMAGED HAIR

Ingredients:

4 Tablespoons Avocado oil

2 Tablespoons Castor oil

1/2 Cup Coconut oil

20 drops Rosemary essential oil

Methods:

1. Mix the entire ingredients in a covered jar.

2. Shake the mixture thoroughly.

Application:

• Scoop up with a fingertip.

• Rub it from the roots of the hair to the tips and scalp thoroughly.

• Allow sitting overnight.

• Shampoo and rinse well.

Storage: Store in a dry, cool place.

Shelf life: Not more two applications.

GRAY HAIR TREATMENT

The following homemade organic recipes will help in delaying gray hair. These treatments are designed to either delay early gray hair or to cover it. Immediately you discovered the gray hair has started growing, apply the organic herbs and oils to delay or cover the gray hair.

Benefits of Gray Hair Treatment

1. Helps in the delaying of gray hair.

2. They will bring back the natural color of the hair without using chemical-based hair care products.

3. It helps to prevent hair loss.

Note that treatment can be done 2-3 times per week.

Coco Curry Oil

Ingredients:

2 Cups Coconut oil

Bunches of Curry leaves

Methods:

1. Wash and air dry the curry leaves to get rid of moisture.

2. Pour water into a double boiler and boil the water.

3. Reduce the heat to low to simmer the water.

4. Pour both the coconut oil and curry leaves in a heatproof container.

5. Allow the mixture to infuse for some hours and stir occasionally.

6. Allow cooling for some minutes.

Application:

• Apply the infused oil to the scalp.

• Massage gently on the scalp.

• Allow it to sit overnight or a few hours.

• Rinse and shampoo the hair.

Storage: Store in a cool, dry place.

Shelf life: If there is no moisture, it can last for more than two years.

Aloe Vera Mask

Ingredient:

Aloe Vera (fresh)

Methods:

1. Cut the Aloe Vera plant.

2. Scrape off the Aloe Vera gel.

Application:

• Rub the Aloe Vera gel gently on the scalp directly.

• Massage it evenly from the roots to the tips of the hair.

Storage: Store in a fridge.

Shelf life: Can last up to 6 months.

Ingredients:

Bunch of Henna leaves

2 Cups Sesame oil

Methods:

1. Wash and air dry the henna leaves to remove the moisture.

2. Pour water into a double boiler and boil the water.

3. Reduce the heat to low to simmer the water.

4. Pour both the sesame oil and henna leaves in a heatproof container.

5. Allow the mixture to infuse for some hours and stir occasionally.

6. Allow cooling for some minutes.

Application:

• Apply the henna infused oil to the scalp.

• Massage gently on the scalp.

• Allow it to sit overnight or a few hours.

• Rinse and shampoo the hair.

Storage: Store in a covered jar and place in a dry, cool place.

Shelf life: Can last up to one year without moisture.

HAIR LOSS TREATMENT

This treatment is about making use of organic oil-based recipes to get back hair growth and stimulate the hair follicle.

Benefits of Hair Loss treatment

1. Ability to stimulate blood circulation in the scalp.

2. Aids the hair follicle for hair growth.

3. Restore the luster in the hair.

4. Ability to prevent excessive shedding of hair.

Note that this treatment can be done as often as necessary.

HAIR LOSS TREATMENT RECIPES

COCO HIBISCUS HAIR OIL

Ingredients:

1/2 Cup Coconut oil

4 Hibiscus leaves

1/2 Cup Badam oil

1 Cup Hibiscus leaves

Methods:

1. Wash the hibiscus leaves to remove the moisture.

2. Sun-dry the hibiscus to get rid of any moisture.

3. Pour the hibiscus flower and leaves in a heatproof bowl.

4. Add badam oil and coconut oil.

5. Transfer the heatproof bowl on a double boiler.

6. Set the fire in low heat.

7. Infuse both the oils and hibiscus for 10 minutes.

8. Strain the oil and pour it into a bottle.

Application:

• Take the amount needed for the hair.

• Warm it slightly.

• Apply the warm oil from the roots to the tips of the hair.

• Rub the scalp for few minutes to enhance the blood circulation.

• Allow sitting overnight.

• Rinse and shampoo the hair the next day.

Storage: Keep in a jar.

Shelf life: Should not be for more than one year with no moisture.

GINGER HAIR OIL

Ingredients:

2 Tablespoons of Ginger (grated)

1 Cup Olive oil

6 drops Rosemary essential oil

Methods:

1. Heat the Olive oil on low heat.

2. Add the ginger and allow boiling until the moisture evaporates.

3. Allow the mixture to cool.

4. Strain the oil and pour it into a dark glass

bottle.

5. Then add rosemary oil.

6. Shake the mixture very well.

Application:

• Rub the mixture from the roots to the tips of hair up to the scalp.

• Massage the scalp gently.

• Allow sitting for more than 15 minutes.

• Use lukewarm water to rinse and apply mild shampoo.

• If there is irritation, shampoo the hair well to get rid of oil.

Storage: Store in a dark, cool place.

Shelf life: Must not be more than two weeks.

Chapter 8

HOME CHART GUIDE (DIY)

This chapter will put you on the road to how to start making your recipe. In the earlier chapters, you have been shown more about essential oils, herbs, and carrier oils. With the step by step guide included in this chapter, you will be able to prepare your concoction.

The tables below illustrate the benefits each oil will give your hair.

Herbs and Essential oils

Herbs	Hair Loss	Body/ Luster	Oily Hair	Scalp	Dry/ Damage	Graying	Dandruff
Aloe Vera	Yes	Yes	No	Yes	Yes	No	No
Amla	Yes	No	No	Yes	Yes	No	No
Aritha	Yes	Yes	No	yes	No	No	Yes
Basil	Yes	Yes	No	Yes	Yes	No	No
Bhringraj	Yes	No	No	No	Yes	Yes	Yes
Black Tea	No	No	Yes	No	No	Yes	No
Burdoch	No	No	No	Yes	Yes	No	Yes
Calendula	No	No	Yes	No	Yes	Yes	No
Chamomile	No	No	Yes	Yes	No	Yes	No
Curry	No	No	No	No	No	Yes	No
Henna	No	Yes	No	No	Yes	Yes	No
Lavender	Yes	Yes	No	Yes	No	No	Yes
Nettle	Yes	Yes	Yes	YEs	Yes	No	Yes
Peppermint	Yes	Yes	Yes	No	No	No	No
Rosemary	Yes	Yes	Yes	Yes	Yes	No	No
Yucca Root	Yes	No	No	Yes	Yes	No	Yes

Carrier oils

Carrier Oil	Nourish	Scalp	Oily	Shiny	Dry/Damage	Gray	Hair Loss	Conditions
Jojoba Oil	Yes	No	No	No	yes	No	No	No
Coconut Oi	Yes	Yes	No	Yes	yes	No	No	Yes
Olive Oil	No	Yes		Yes	No	No	No	No
Sweet Almo	No	Yes	Yes		No	Yes	Yes	Yes
Apricot	No	Yes	Yes	No	No	No	Yes	No
Avocado	Yes	Yes	No	No	Yes	No	No	Yes
Argan	No	No	No	Yes	Yes	No	No	Yes
Grapeseed	Yes	Yes	Yes	Yes	No	No	No	No
Hazel Nut	Yes	Yes	No	No	Yes	No	No	No
Sesame	Yes	Yes	No	No	Yes	Yes	No	No

DIY PROCEDURE

Below is a step by step guide on how to have homemade infused oil.

1. Choose Treatment:

The first step is to choose the type of treatment

to be prepared. Is it pre-poo, conditioner, or damaged hair oil?

Which of deep conditioner, pre-poo, or light conditioner treatment is to start with? Remember that deep conditioner treatment will treat scalp and some other hair problems.

2. Choose Herbs and Essential oil

There are many herbs to choose from, so it is better to choose the one that will address your required treatment.

You can combine essential oil and fresh herbs to the recipe you desire, only remember to dilute both with a carrier oil.

To have a deep conditioner choose Aloe Vera to combine with burdock essential oil.

To have light conditioner treatment choose Yucca root to combine with rosemary or lavender essential oil. Yucca root contains cleansing properties suitable for the hair.

3. Choose Carrier oil

The main function of carrier oil is to dilute essential oil extracted from herbs. It will reduce the harshness of the herbs.

Coconut oil is best to be mixed with Aloe Vera as part of the conditioning ingredients. Coconut oil has the characteristic to treat scalp and be able to nourish hair.

For light conditioners, choose sesame oil to dilute the essential oil.

4. Preparing infusion

Whenever the infusion is to be prepared, place

it on extremely low heat so that the oils will not be destroyed.

Make use of a double boiler for the mixture to be steam heated rather than direct heat.

5. Storing the mixture

Make sure you store the mixture in a sterilized covered jar and keep it in a dry, cool place away from being exposed to the sun.

Remember that some mixtures need refrigeration for storage. Use a bowl for deep conditioner so that it will be easier to use fingers to scoop the mix for the application.

Light conditioner can be turned to leave-in conditioner as it can be poured into a spritzer and be carried around and spray when necessary.

6. Apply the mixture

Rub the significant portion to the hair. The more the damage, the more the application required.

CONCLUSION

Haircare is time immemorial.

The hair care industry is enormous, and it's growing every year.

This book has given many herbs, essential oils, and carrier oils to make your hair healthy, improve the blood circulation of the scalp, and stimulate the growth of hair follicles. The recipes in this guide are to activate the dermal papilla in the hair follicles and enhance scalp metabolism to aids the natural hair growth.

Another objective of this book is to address the challenges of looking for herbal hair products that are not expensive and can be made at home. The information in this book aims to expose people to how to use herbal products coupled with different ingredients that can be found easily in the kitchen or at the supermarket stores.

You have read this guide on "Homemade Herbal Hair Oil Infusions: Easy Guide to Herbal Hair Oil Infusions Recipes for Hair Growth, Dry/Damaged Hair, Dandruff and Healthy Scalp," the next step is for you to use the tips given to know what works for you and not. In as much you are careful with the recipes and blends of essential oils with other ingredients presented in the book, you are assured that you will achieve the benefits associated with healthy hair and scalp.

Please buy your oils from reputable suppliers or

store, and take time to check the reviews before bringing out your wallet. So many companies only supply synthetic essential oils that they claimed are pure and organic.

Thanks You.